Chicken

A Quick Guide on Chicken Breeds for Beginners

Norman Nelson

PUBLISHED BY:
Norman Nelson
Copyright © 2013

Table of Contents

Chapter 1: Introduction

History

The first chickens kept by man were the Red Jungle Fowl. These birds were related to the pheasant family and some were cross bred with the Grey Jungle Fowl. It is found in South India, where it is cross bred with domestic chickens. It is also found in Southern China, Malaysia, Philippines, Indonesia, and certain islands of Hawaii, Christmas Islands and Mariana Islands in the NW Pacific.

These chickens have been raised and kept by people for at least 5,000 years. They were mainly kept for cock fighting and later for meat and eggs. Their domestication began in Asia and spread around the world. In 3000 BC, the chicken was introduced to Europe, Ukraine, Greece, Romania and Turkey. In 1000 BC, the chicken found its way to several parts of the Middle East and Western Europe. Breeding was done extensively in Roman times but was reduced in the middle ages. The Indian Red Jungle Fowl was bred at first for cock fights but later started to be bred for meat and eggs. Selective breeding started in the Roman Empire from which many domestic breeds are now seen.

A Chicken's Life Cycle

The chicken's life cycle begins with the fertilization of the egg by the rooster; the hen lays the egg and sits on it for a period of 21 days. After this period of time, the chick break out of the shell and a chick is born. The chick then grows and is ready to lay eggs in 4 to 6 months, depending on the breed. The lighter egg laying breeds will start laying before the heavier breeds. The cycle then starts again.

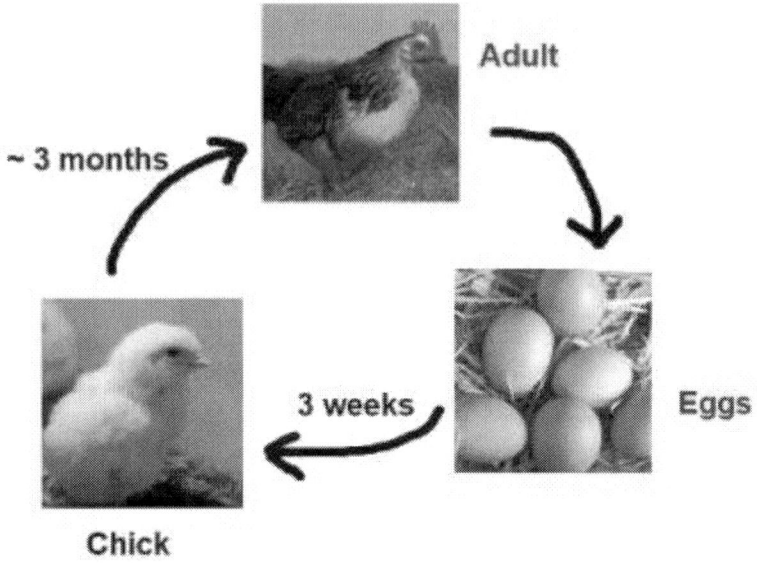

~ 3 months

Adult

Eggs

3 weeks

Chick

Typical Differences between a Rooster and a Hen

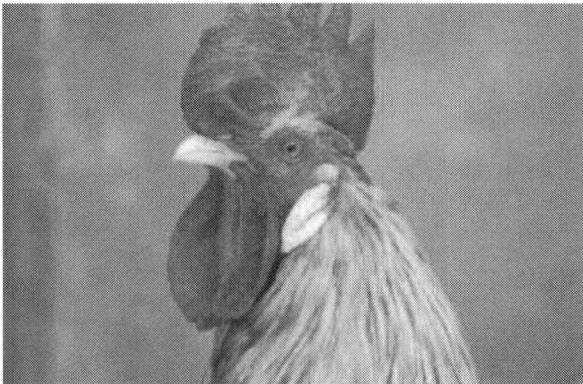

Rooster

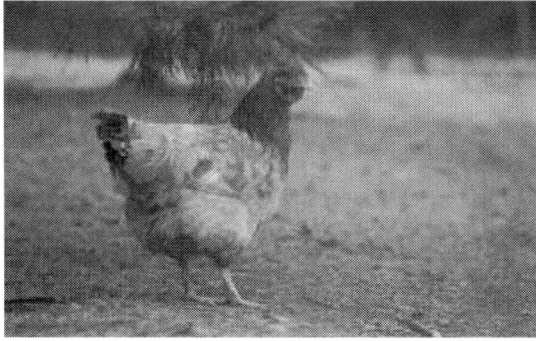
Hen

As with most birds, the rooster has more elaborate feathers than the hen. The illustration shows the bigger comb and wattles of the rooster, compared to the hen. The feathers on the neck known as the saddle feathers are larger and often have more color than the hen. The rooster's tail feathers are his trademark, arching up and over to form a colorful cascade. The color will depend on the breed. The rooster's claws are usually longer than the hen and will have a spur on their foot to protect the flock and fight for their supremacy as the head rooster of the flock. The rooster is usually a bigger bird than the hen. He will also have a characteristic call known as crowing. Their penis is situated internally, which is why they need to angle themselves on the hen's back to mate with them. Both hens and roosters have a cloaca, which they used in mating.

The hen on the other hand has a smaller comb and wattles. Some breeds do not have a comb. She is less colorful and her feathers are shorter. Her color is often to help her become better camouflaged as she is the only one that looks after the eggs and small chicks. Internally they will have a reproductive system that will be geared for creating eggs. They have a universal opening for eggs, stool and urine called the cloaca.

Chapter 2: Anatomy of Chicken

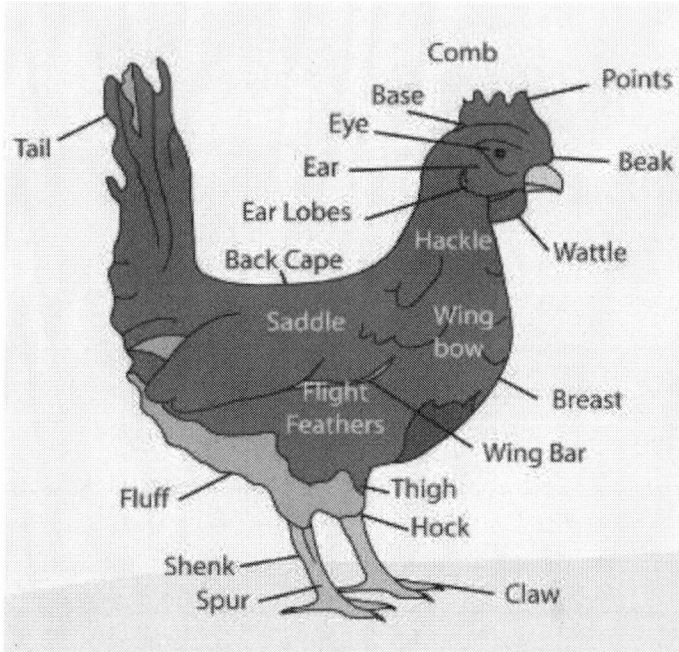

The illustration shows the parts of the chicken that you should know about. The breast and wings are known as white meat. The breast of the chicken is known for its flavor and tenderness and is the most expensive cut of the bird. The wings do not have much meat and are generally a cheaper cut of meat. The dark meat is the thighs and legs of the bird. The meat is still flavorful but not as tender.

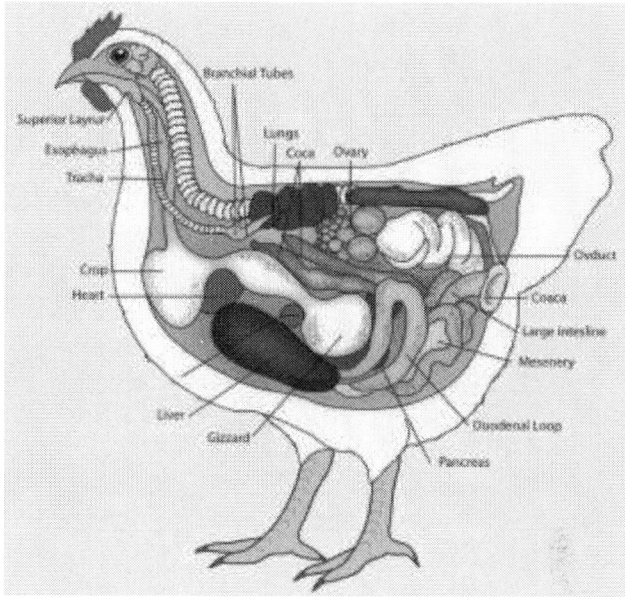

Parts of a Chicken Head

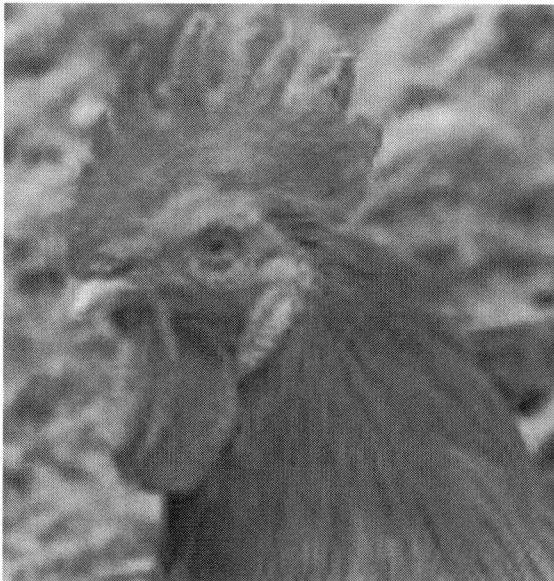

The chicken's head will tell you a lot about their overall health.

Comb: This is the fleshy appendage that grows on top of the bird's head. It is sometimes a regular comb, or a rose comb and is sometimes absent in some breeds of a hen. They are usually red or pink. Roosters have more prominent combs.

Beak: It is usually predominantly yellow; with some breeds like the illustration above has some black markings. It is of medium length and sturdy as the chicken is an omnivore.

Eye: A healthy bird will have prominent bright eyes. A chicken will need to pivot its head to see things from the side. This is why a chicken will often look at you with its head slightly tilted. Chickens see well as long as it is daylight but do not see well at night. This means that they need a secure place to sleep at night.

Ear: Birds do not have external ears like mammals, but have internal ears. They have two ear lobes, one on each side of the head. Some breeds will have little tufts of feathers around this area.

Wattles: These are two appendages that will hang below the beak on each side of the face. They are fleshy like the comb and will be pink or red according to the comb of the bird.

Crop: All birds will have this on the throat above the breast. This acts as the teeth of the chicken and requires grit or little stones to help grind down the food for the bird.

Parts of the Wing

It is good to know the parts of a chicken's wing. They are a popular part of the chicken to eat and it is good to know about the different parts that can get injured. First there is the wing shoulder where the chicken's body joins with the wing. This is called the drumette when you eat wings. There are a number of different types of feathers that cover this part of the chicken. Then there is the mid joint of the wing, which is often called the wingette or flat when you eat it. The wing tip is usually removed before you cook this part of the chicken. It consists of long feathers known as the primary ones. These are the feathers that are trimmed when you clip the wings of a chicken.

Parts of Single Feather

This illustration can be found at
http://www.backyardchickens.com/a/my-feather-anatomy-guide

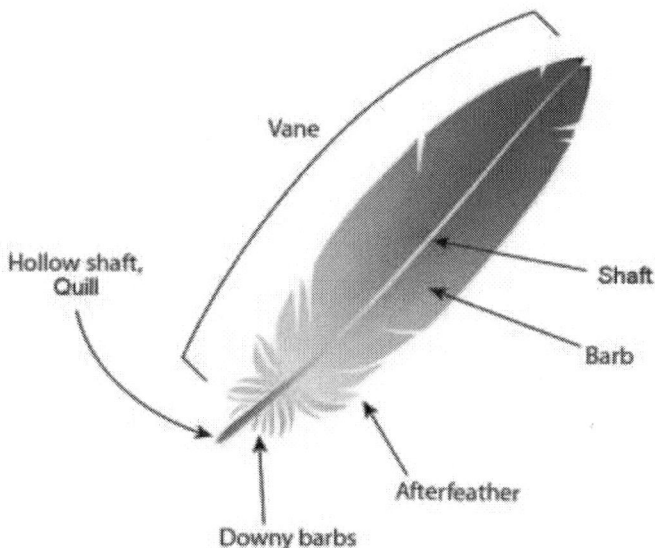

Vane

Hollow shaft, Quill

Shaft

Barb

Afterfeather

Downy barbs

A chicken basic feather structure looks like this. They are termed hard or soft feathered birds according to the stiffness of the shaft. For example the English Game Bird breed of chicken is referred to as a hard feathered breed as the shaft of the feathers is very stiff and the feathers grow close together. The Japanese Silkie is a soft feathered bird as the shaft is less stiff and the breed is characterized as a round, soft variety. Of course there are a number of different patterns which will depend on the breed of chicken. Most chickens are barbed varieties, with the exception of the Silkies. The Standard of Perfection is used to define different breeds.

Different Types of Chicken Combs

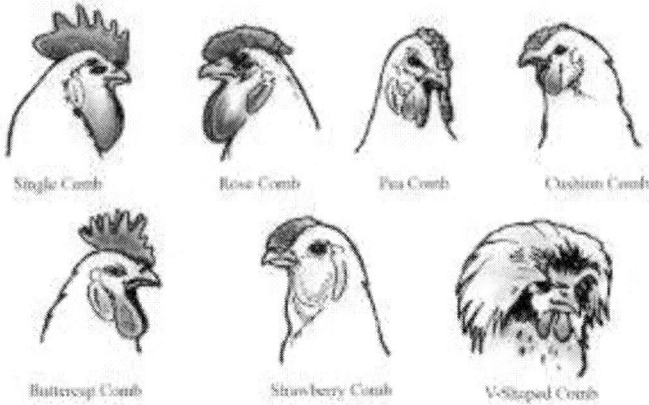

Single Comb Rose Comb Pea Comb Cushion Comb

Buttercup Comb Strawberry Comb V-Shaped Comb

There are about 9 different types of combs that you will find in chickens, 7 of which are illustrated here. These differences will depend upon the age, sex and breed of the chicken. Roosters will always have a larger and brighter colored comb than the hens.

The network of blood vessels in the comb and wattles keeps the chickens cool during the summer. The blood gets cooler as it circulates through them. This in turn will decrease the temperature of the chicken. The comb is also a way of attracting a mate. The rooster or hen with the brightest and biggest comb will become the dominant ones of the flock. The growth of the comb in small chicks is a sign of a pullet or cockerel, so breeders watch for this.

Single Comb
It is the most common form of comb in American breeds. It grows on top of the chicken's head, in a straight line from the beak to the back of the head. It is smooth and soft to touch. The comb itself consists of 5 to 6 points and a thicker portion behind called the blade. It is usually

red and can hang over one side on the hens. Examples of breeds with single comb are Rhode Island Reds and Leghorns.

Rose Comb

This type of comb resembles a tube with a spike at the end. The front two thirds of the comb have small bumps on it. Some breeds like Rhode Island Reds and Leghorns can also have these types of combs; other breeds include Hamburg and Wyandotte.

Spiked Rose Comb

This is similar to the rose comb but will have a longer spike at the back of the comb.

Pea Comb

This type of comb has three ridges or points and is medium in size. Breeds like Araucanas and Brahmins have these types of combs.

Cushion Comb

This style of comb is a round small comb with no points or ridges. Breeds like Chanteclers will have this type of comb.

Buttercup Comb

This comb forms a circle on top of the chicken's head. It can be seen in Sicilian Buttercup varieties of chicken. It looks similar to the single comb in that it has points.

Strawberry Comb

This type of comb can be seen Yokohamas and Malay breeds. It is similar to the cushion comb except that it has bumps like a strawberry.

V-Shaped Comb

This comb has 2 points that start at the base of the bird's beak and extend to the back of its head. There is often a crest of feathers in the middle. Breeds like Polish and Houdans display this sort of crest.

Walnut

This is a medium size comb. It has furrows like a walnut shell. Japanese Silkies have this type of comb. It is a cross between a pea and rose comb.

Different Kinds of Chicken Plumages

Different colored plumage, or feathers, indicates different breeds of chicken. Due to sophisticated methods of breeding many variations of feather markings can be seen in chickens. Here are a few:

Barring

This refers to the horizontal stripes on a chicken comprised of 2 colors, an example of a regular stripe in the Plymouth Rock, which is often known as the Barred Rock due to its markings. An irregular stripe when one color is dominant is known as a cuckoo bar and can be found in breeds like the Dominique and Hollander.

Frizzle Feathers

These types of feathers are also known as twisted ones. The web and shaft of the feather are twisted creating the frizzle varieties.

Laced Feathers

This pattern has a contrasting color on the border on the web of the wing. This marking will be found on most blue breeds of chicken and also some varieties of Polish and Cochin breeds.

Single Lace

This pattern of plumage is seen by the single contrasting color on the border of the web of the wing. Laced Hamburg varieties and Laced Polish breeds will exhibit these markings.

Double Lace

This marking will be seen by a double boarder around the wing web. It is often black or a contrasting color. This can be seen in Laced varieties

Mottled Feather
This pattern consists of white tips on the feathers. Not every feather has this marking. Examples of breeds that have these markings are Anconas and Houdans.

Penciling
This can be seen by crosswise stripes on hens like the penciled Hamburg breed. These stripes can also go the full length of the feather. This is seen in the Wyandotte and Cochin varieties. The Standard of perfection specifies that there should be at least 3 pencil markings on every feather of the thigh, back, wing bows, body and breast plumage.

Peppered Feathers
These are small black dots that are found in the feather marking of a chicken. They are considered a defect by the American Standard of Perfection, the book by which breeders judge breeds of chicken.

Spangled Feathers
The wing tips of these birds have a tear drop of black or white at the wing tip. Speckled Sussex and Hamburg varieties of breeds display these markings.

Splashed Feathers
These markings are displayed by different splashes of contrasting color on the bird's plumage. This creates a mottled look.

Blue Fowls
Blue fowls have been especially bred for their bluish color. They can range from black with a bluish tinge to a light slate grey. The Andalusia breed of chicken is the original Blue Chicken breed but will not always

produce 100% blue chickens. It is quite hard to breed blue colored chickens in larger quantities.

Avian Genetics Determination

How Can I Determine the Sex of a Baby Chick?

There are a number of tests that can be done for determining the sex of the chicken. It is quite difficult to do this if you are new to chickens. The best thing to do when you go out to purchase your chicks is to take an experienced chicken breeder with you. If you do this you will be able to do the butt bump test. This is a test that hatcheries and professionals use. They gently squeeze the chick to find out if it has a bump at the butt, if they do this indicates that the chick is a cockerel, or young rooster. An absence of the bump means that the chick is a pullet, or young hen. If you are not familiar with chickens, it is wise to let someone who is more experienced to do this to avoid harming or hurting the chick.

As the chicks grow you will find that the roosters develop a bigger comb and wattles than the hens. You will be able to determine this when the chicks are about 6 to 8 weeks old. With some breeds you can do the wing test. Females grow feathers faster than the males so will have uneven feathers on their wings. Both these tests will be for older chicks.

With some breeds you can tell their sex by color. This is simple to do with the Red Star Sex Link as the cockerels will be yellow and the pullets will be red in color. Some breeds will have slightly lighter chicks as males and darker ones as females.

Components of Chicken Chromosomes and Chicken Chromosomes Structure

Chickens have pairs of 78 chromosomes, with the majority being microchromosomes. There are 2 ways that scientists classify them. Some say that they have 8 pairs of macrochromosomes, 1 pair of sex chromosomes and 32 pairs of microchromosomes. The "International Chicken Genome Sequencing Consortium" classifies the chicken chromosomes into 5 pairs of macrochromosomes, 5 pairs of chromosomes that are intermediate and 28 pairs of microchromosomes. These microchromosomes form $1/3^{rd}$ of the size of the genome and have a much higher gene density.

Because the majority of the chicken's chromosomes are microchromosomes they have the capacity to be very diverse genetically. The chromosome 16 in chickens which is a microchromosome is one of the most diverse genetic chromosomes in some breeds of chicken. These components of chicken chromosomes account for the many different breeds of chicken.

Chapter 3: Chicken Breeding

In chicken breeding, you want to preserve the strong qualities of the flock and if possible improve their productive qualities. These different techniques will help you understand how to achieve these two goals.

Chicken Breeding Techniques

Grading

This is how a flock can be improved by modifying traits. The chicken is graded for characteristics that the breeder wants. For example if they are looking for egg laying traits they will grade the chickens to be breed for egg laying traits and choose the best ones for breeding the best egg layers.

This is done by breeding with different strains and types of chicken which have strong characteristics that you want bred into your flock. Six to eight generations of breeding will be counted as pure stock. A flock can be modified and strengthened for different purposes by this method. Once the right traits have been established the birds are often returned to the flock and the rolling method can be used.

Rolling Mating

This method of mating is also known as 'The Old Farmer's Method." Young cockerels are mated with mature hens and young pullets are mated with mature roosters. This method requires two flocks one for the mature birds and one for the pullets and cockerels. The birds are culled at the end of the breeding season, so that only the best birds are used for breeding and the flock is kept at a proper number. This method works well in that you will find few birds that are related to each other. This allows you to keep a stronger flock.

Single Mating

This is when the standard of breeding only requires the same genetic traits from the male and female. Therefore you need just one pen of birds and the pair only has to mate once. The rooster and hen are both exhibition birds.

Out and Out Mating

This form of mating is when you bring a new rooster from an outside source each year. This method was used with cross breeds but is also used for pure bred chickens. This is done to stop weakening of the flock by too much family interbreeding. However, it can also have its disadvantages. The strong traits of the first breeding may not be present with a different rooster as each rooster comes with different traits.

Clan Mating

This is when the flock is divided into families. Each family will be bred separately and either the rooster or hen's lines will be used. The roosters and hens of the same clan are not used for breeding. Often 3 sets of clans can be used, when using the maternal lines. The birds should be identified and also the eggs. A rooster can be used to mate with the hens of the all 3 clans. Chicken fanciers use this method.

Family mating

This is when a pair creates pullets and cockerels. These sons and daughters will be allowed to mate with family members. The genetic lines are preserved but sometimes you will experience certain family weaknesses which can worsen with family breeding.

Out-Cross breeding

This form of breeding is using a new rooster every year to fertilize the hens. The rooster will not be the same breed as the hens so that cross breeding is practiced.

Cross Breeding

Cross breeding is when birds of different breeds are mated to produce certain characteristics and enhance traits. This is practiced to produce the best egg layers or meat producing chickens and sometimes results in problems for the birds. The birds that are cross bred for fast growth can experience chronic hunger and also skeletal problems. These hybrid breeds are often kept in bad conditions and treated like machines. Now steps are being taken to improve these chickens' welfare.

Chicken fanciers also cross breed chickens to get beautiful birds for show. An example of this would be the English bantam breed the Sebright. This bird has been especially bred for the pattern of its plumage. It is quite hard to breed duplicates of this beautiful plumage.

Line Breeding

This is when the same pair of birds is used for a number of years to breed stock birds.

This form of breeding was perfected by the "cockers" or fighting cock experts. If they found a pair of chickens that produced good performers in the pit then they would use them for as long as 5 years. Free range birds were generally used for breeding, so that the chickens were able to reach optimum strength and prowess.

In-Breeding

In-breeding is when the breeder uses the stock they have. They will grade the birds and only use chickens that produce the traits they were looking for. Outside birds were not used for this purpose. It is a form of breeding that was practiced by those interested in fighting cocks. They breed only from the best and most vigorous birds in the flock. This required ruthless culling and using the youngest birds in the stock. They sought out the pairs that produced the best performers in the pit. This meant that breeds were kept relatively pure, as they did not use out breeding or cross breeding much, except to improve the vigor and endurance of the bird.

Artificial Insemination

The semen is collected by massaging the abdomen of the rooster and applying a little pressure. Freshly collected semen is best for artificial insemination. Frozen sperm is not as fertile as fresh sperm. This method will increase the fertility of the eggs, but requires some skill so is best practiced by someone with experience.

In order to collect the maximum amount of sperm from the rooster the less stress the bird experiences the more you can collect. If there is more of a struggle to capture and restrain the rooster, less semen will be collected.

The advantages of artificial insemination are:

- Roosters with good linage can fertilize particular hens easily.

- Fewer males can be used to fertilize the hens, which work out to more efficient feed to chicken ratio.
- The recording of pedigree is more accurate.
- 5% to 10% increase in fertility can be achieved
- Large roosters can be paired with smaller hens, or pairing of a smaller rooster with a larger hen can be done, using artificial insemination.

Sex-Link Cross

This is when breeders make use of the sex chromosomes in the hen and roster. These birds are specially hybrid to produce different colors for pullets, cockerels and chicks.

Sex link cross breeds are breed so that the cockerel chicks are a different color from the pullets. This makes it easier to differentiate between the sexes when they are chicks. The basic colors of the chicken are red, or gold and black. These Sex-Link chickens are hybrid so will not breed true. Some of the most popular are:

- **Black Sex-Link Cross:** These chickens are a cross between a Barred Rock hen with a Rhode Island Red or New Hampshire rooster. The cockerels and pullets will both have black down but the cockerels will have a white dot on the top of their head.

- **Red-Sex Link Cross:** This is a cross of a Rhode Island Red or New Hampshire rooster and either a White Rock, White Laced Wyandotte, or Rhode Island White hen. The pullets are buff with red and the cockerels are white.

- **Fast Feathering Growth**
  This is used to differentiate between the sexes of broiler types of sex link chicks. The difference in sex can be seen by the different growth of the primary and covert feathers in chicks

that are 1 to 3 days old. The primary feathers are long and covert ones short in this variety.

- **Slow Feathering Growth:** The covert feathers are long and primary ones short on slow feathered varieties. The sex of the chicks can be seen from this in chicks that are 1 to 3 days old. The males will be slow in feathering and the females grown their feathers fast.

Purpose of Breeding a Chicken

There are a number of reasons that breeders work with chickens. Firstly, they may want to improve the traits in a chicken and secondly the breeder may want to make the chicken more attractive.

- **Dual Purpose:** Dual purpose birds are good for meat and egg laying. When breeding these chickens the breeder will look for good egg laying traits as well as fast growth. They will also look for flavor and the size of the chicken. To enhance these qualities they will use these breeding techniques. Grading will be used to bring out the best traits in the bird. Crossbreeding can also be used to improve the traits. These birds tend to be a little heavier to accommodate meat traits. They will also be cross bred with birds of good egg laying qualities. Inline breeding techniques will keep the traits of the chicken. Examples of dual purpose breeds are Plymouth Rocks and Rhode Island Reds.

- **Egg Layer:** The birds will be bred in the same way as above. However instead of looking for meat characteristics the breeder will just look for better egg laying traits. They can be crossbred to bring out the best egg laying traits and graded. Once strong egg laying traits are established inline breeding can be practiced, using the best pairs of birds. The egg laying breeds are usually lighter birds like Leghorns. The Aracuna chicken lays colored eggs and is a fun and profitable laying chicken to keep. Sometimes when you cross breed one of these birds with another good laying breed you will get a good laying chicken which lays colored eggs.

- **Meat Production:** The breeder will be looking for fast growing, heavier birds. They will use crossbreeding techniques and hybrid breeds. Genetic engineering has been used for this type of breeding, as it is a huge part of the chicken industry. Large birds like Jersey Giants have been created. Chickens breed for meat are ready for the table in 5 to 8 weeks.

- **Ornamental Purpose:** In order to create the most beautiful breeds of birds, cross breeding was practiced. An example of years of painstaking breeding is the bantam Sebright chicken. This bird is difficult to duplicate because of the breeding techniques.

- **Competition Purpose:** The first competition breeders were the "cockers" who were interested in cock fights. They used a 6 point method of breeding. They used only the best birds to breed from and culled ruthlessly. Once they found a good pair that bred the birds they were looking for, they used them for 5 years. They kept their breeding stock young and kept detailed records of their results. Their chickens were always free range which helped the birds keep its optimum health and strength. This was in fact the ultimate inline breeding technique.

Chicken Breeds Size

When the average person thinks about chickens they often think about the standard size chickens but there are other sizes available.

- **Bantam:** These are small breeds of chicken that are often kept for pets or exhibition. These birds are about ¼ the size of standard chickens. Many people who raise bantams will take them to exhibitions. Especially the true bantam variety of Sebrights which are beautiful birds. Bantams make good pets as they are small and easier to keep than the large chickens. If you have a smaller space then these birds are good to keep. Most of them are not quite as docile as their standard counterparts. However, Japanese Silkie bantams are still docile and make good pets. They are also good brooders which make them good for breeding. These birds are not usually bred for eggs and meat.

- **Large Fowl:** These birds are standard size chickens and can be bred for meat and eggs. Some people also use them for shows and exhibition purposes. Now there are breeds that have been created, like the Jersey Giant breed that are larger than standard birds and are bred for meat. Meat varieties of birds are heavier than the egg layers and are bred for their fast growth. These birds can be ready for the table by 5 to 8 weeks old. The chickens are also bred for flavor. Some of the popular meat or broilers are Orpingtons and Cornish breeds.

APA/ABA Chicken Breeds Class

This is how chickens are classed by the APA/ABA

American Breeds

These are those that have originated in the US. Many of these breeds were developed for their egg laying prowess as well as their meat. This makes them dual purpose birds. Examples of popular American class breeds are:

- **Plymouth Rocks:** This is a dual purpose breed that lays brown eggs.

- **Wyandottes:** This is another dual purpose chicken that will lay brown eggs
.

- **Rhode Island Reds:** This breed is an all time favorite and is a dual purpose bird. It lays good sized brown eggs.

- **Jersey Giants:** These are large birds that were bred for meat. However they also lay brown eggs.

- **New Hampshires:** These are dual purpose chickens and lay brown eggs.

Asiatic Breeds

Many of these breeds originated in China. These birds are often breed for dual purpose, meat and eggs. Some are also breed for exhibition purposes. Examples of these breeds are:

- **Brahmas:** This is a heavy breed of chicken and can be used for both eggs and meat. The breed is hardy in cold winters. It has feathered legs and feet.

- **Langshans:** This is another dual purpose breed that originated in China.

English Breeds

This class of chicken is breed in the UK. They were bred primarily for eggs and meat. Cock fighting was popular and led to some breeds like the Cornish breed. Some birds were also bred for exhibition purposes.

- **Dorkings:** It is a heavy breed that is breed for meat and exhibition purposes.

- **Redcaps:** This breed is also known as Derbyshire Redcap. It was created as a dual purpose breed, but is now used for its white eggs.

- **Cornish:** This breed was bred by cockers for cock fights. They were bred in Cornwall. It is a heavy bird and is now breed for meat. The birds have pea combs and red ear lobes. The chicken has widespread thick legs and come in 3 colors, white laced with chestnut, chestnut with double lacing of greenish black, and blue. They often go by the name of Indian Game birds. They do become tame quite easily and are not as aggressive as other Game birds.

- **Orpingtons:** Is a heavy breed that also lays well. It has light brown eggs and is used for both eggs and meat.

- **Sussex:** This is a heavy breed of bird which is used for the dual purpose of eggs and meat.

- **Australorps:** Are usually black heavy breeds and were imported to the UK in the 1920's from Australia. They have serrated single combs and are docile in nature. They are good layers of tinted brown eggs. They are dual purpose birds and are a good breed for beginners.

Mediterranean Breeds

These breeds of chicken are those that originated from countries that border the Mediterranean Sea which included Italy and Spain. Many of these breeds were bred for eggs and a number of them are good layers of white eggs. They are often lighter breeds and do not brood. The majorities of these birds are quite flighty by nature and do not make good pets. These birds have single or rose combs and clean legs. Here are some examples:

- **Leghorns:** Are light breeds of bird that are exceptionally good at laying eggs. The white ones are used commercially. They lay white eggs.

- **Minorcas:** These chickens are similar to the Leghorn except that they are black with white earlobes. They are good layers of large white eggs.

- **Spanish:** These birds are characterized by their white faces and long white earlobes. They lay white eggs.

- **Andalusians:** They are the original blue chickens which have been breed with other breeds to create other blue varieties of chickens. It also lays white eggs.

- **Anconas:** Are often black with a white V-shape on each feather. It lays white eggs.

- **Sicilian buttercups:** These are a rare breed of chicken. The hen is mottled and the rooster a rich red brown with black tail feathers. They lay a few white eggs.

- **Catalanas:** Are buff colored chickens breed for meat and white eggs.

Continental Breeds

These are breeds that originated from the north of Europe and were bred for meat and eggs. Many of this class originated in Holland. Examples of these are:

- **Hamburgs:** These are a light breed of egg laying birds. They are also ornamental and can be used for exhibition purposes.

- Barnevelder: This is a dual purpose bird that comes in a variety of colors. It lays brown eggs.

Feather Legged

There are a number of feather legged chickens. They are often used for exhibition purposes. Examples of these are:

- Belgian D'Uccle: This is a bantam variety of breed and can also come in a bearded breed. It is most commonly used for exhibition purposes.

- Brahma: This is a heavy bred that comes in a variety of colors. They lay brown eggs.

- Cochin: This Chinese breed comes in a variety of colors. It has a pleasant personality and is a fluffy variety of chicken.

- Langshan: This is a rare breed from China. They are white, black and blue and lay brown eggs.

- Sultans: These are white birds with crests, beards and feathered feet and legs. They are used for exhibition purposes.

Polish Breeds

These birds are a light variety with a crest on top of their heads. They come in a variety of colors and some are bearded, others are not. They can be solid black with a white crest or solid blue with a white crest. They come in white, silver laced, buff laced, gold laced, cuckoo and spangled. They are often used as exhibition birds and are some of the oldest breeds of chicken. Despite their name they do not originate in Poland but in Europe, England, Holland or France. They do not see too well because of their crest and have a tendency to panic easily. When breeding these birds you can mate a frizzle with a plain bird and get both types but do not pair 2 frizzles together or you will have a chicken without feathers. Special care is needed not to get them wet as their crests take time to dry. Some people will dry their crests with a hair dryer before the chicken sleeps, as they are quite susceptible to colds. It is wise to have nipple watering dispensers rather than regular ones so the bird's crest does not stop them from drinking.

French Breeds

These breeds originated in France. Many of these birds were bred for meat, but can also be used for eggs as well. The crested varieties can also be used for exhibition purposes. Here are some examples.

- **Faverolles:** This breed is another dual purpose chicken which is good for meat and egg laying production.

- **Houdan:** This breed was originally bred for meat but is now used for exhibitions, as it is really a light breed of chicken.

- **Creve-Coeur:** This breed was bred for meat and is crossed with the Dorking to make it bigger.

- **La Fleche:** This heavy breed is an old one from France.

- **Modern Game Breed:** Originally this breed of chicken was inbred by cockers who bred it for cock fights. It was crossed with the Old English Game and Malay. This chicken is a tall bird with long legs and a longer neck. It is now bred for exhibition purposes. They are smaller birds and become tame easily, which means that they make good pets for the backyard flock owner.

Oriental Breeds

These breeds often originated in China. They are often unusual birds and breed for exhibition purposes. Here are some examples:

- **Frizzle:** This breed comes from Asia and is used for exhibition purposes. The bantam is more popular than the standard variety. It is a heavy breed with unusual tight twists on its feathers. Breeding has to be carefully done. You should not mate the same frizzled birds year after year or you will have chickens that do not have many feathers. Instead a new young rooster, with good frizzle, should be paired with the pullets. These breeds are quite good layers of tinted eggs.

- **Silkie:** This breed comes from China and is popular as a pet. Common colors are black and white. They have a cushion style of comb. The male will have a spiked crest and the hen will have a crest like a powder puff.

- **Malay:** The Malay breed is usually bred for meat or exhibition purposes. They have long necks and legs and not very much plumage. They have a walnut comb and were crossed with the Indian Game Bird to produce the Cornish breed. They come in different colors, like the white and spangled one, black, red porcelain and duckwing.

- **Yokomona:** This Japanese breed is bred for exhibition purposes. The tails of the roosters grow to around 2 feet. Japanese breeders have been able to prevent the birds from molting and achieve 3 foot tails on their roosters. Special care must be taken with these exhibition birds. They will need taller coops and higher roosts than other chickens. They will also need to be kept clean.

Bantam Breeds

These are small replicas of standard breeds. They are about ¼ the size of standard birds, which makes them easier to keep in smaller areas. Some breeds can only be found in bantam form like the Sebright breed and are known as true bantams. As well as being used for pets and as small backyard flock these birds are often used for exhibition purposes.

Single Comb Clean Leg

The Single Comb and Clean Leg varieties of chickens are inherent in many breeds. This simply means that these breeds have single large to medium combs. They usually stand upright but can fall over to one side. Clean legs means that these breeds do not have feathers on their feet or legs, which makes them easier to keep clean.

Chapter 4: Chicken Breeds for Egg Production

How to Raise Chickens for Egg Production

It is important to know that chickens do not need a rooster for laying eggs. They will simply not be fertilized. This is useful to know if city ordinances do not allow roosters. Before you start raising a backyard flock for egg production, it is wise to choose the breeds that are known for their egg laying prowess. You should also consider if you will be using your flock to lay eggs for commercial purposes.

The chickens will need a warm, dry and well-ventilated coop. You should make this secure as there are a number of predators who love to eat chickens. Free range birds are better egg layers as they will lead a more natural life and be less inclined to fight and peck at each other. Therefore it is good to attach a run to the coop for your chickens. This should be covered and be well-secured against predators.

The usual cleaning chores apply as the chickens should be kept clean to stay healthy. They will need clean water and food on a daily basis. If you want to breed egg layers you will find that they are not broody and you will have to learn how to use an incubator. However there are breeds that are brooders and they will happily hatch out eggs the natural way. If you choose a broody breed make sure it is a dual purpose bird who will also supply you with eggs. Egg laying chickens will need egg laying feed at 4 months, or you can make your own. Free range birds are best for egg layers as they will be less irritable and will be able to forage. This adds to the nutrition of the egg and happy hens will lay better.

When Should I Start Collecting Eggs?

Hens start to lay between 4 to 6 months. At first the eggs will be small and elongated. The eggs will get larger as they become mature. For commercial purposes it is wise to sell the eggs when they get to normal size but the first eggs can be consumed at home.

Different Size and Weight of Chicken Eggs

Jumbo: More than 2.5 oz.

Extra-large: More 2.25 oz. and less than 2.5 oz.

Large: More than 2 oz. but less than 2.25 oz.

Medium: More than 1.75 oz.

Small: More than 1.5 oz.

Yellow Skinned Chicken Breeds

Anconas

Class & Type: This is a lighter breed of Mediterranean class and used mainly for eggs.

Origin: It originated in the province of Ancona in Italy. The breed was developed using Leghorns and was named after the port city of Ancona. These birds were first exhibited in the UK in 1851. It arrived in the US in 1888.

Colors: It is a mottled bird with black and white coloring.

Sizes: The breed is termed as light and there is a bantam variety available.

Characteristics: It lays white eggs and is bred for egg laying. It is not a good table bird. The breed is a little excitable. It has long wattles and either a single or rose shaped comb. Light colored ones with no white on their fluff are best for egg laying. The breed is termed as soft feathered and lays large white eggs.

Barnevelders

Class & Type: This breed is known as a Continental class and is a heavier breed.

Origin: This breed originated in the Netherlands and they originally came from an area in Holland known as Barnevelder.

Colors: It comes in a variety of colors but for exhibition purposes the colors that are accepted are Blue Double Laced, White Black and Double Laced.

Sizes: It is a medium heavy breed used for both meat and eggs.

Characteristics: It is a heavy breed and has a single comb. They are dual purpose birds that lay large dark brown eggs. These chickens are docile birds which make them ideal for beginners.

Leghorns

Class & Type: This breed is classified as a Mediterranean variety and is a light breed.

Origin: This chicken breed originated in Italy

Colors: There are a number of colors for these birds but white is the most common.

Sizes: They are a light breed and available in standard and bantam.

Characteristics: They are famous for their egg laying prowess. They have big single combs which flop over on one side. The other colors have been developed by breeders around the world. They are quite flighty but their egg laying traits are good for backyard flocks, especially if you want to sell the eggs. They lay extra-large white eggs.

Sicilian Buttercup

Class & Type: This is a Mediterranean class of chicken.

Origin: The breed originated from the island of Sicily.

Colors: They are a rich brown variety.

Sizes: They are a light breed and are available in standard and bantam varieties.

Characteristics: They have clean legs and have a buttercup comb which contributes to their beauty. This breed is not very friendly so it might not be the best choice for the beginner. The roosters are friendlier than the hens. They fly well so the run needs to be covered. They are fair layers of small white eggs. It is a rare breed of chicken.

Welsummers

Class & Type: This breed is termed a Continental class of bird and is a light breed.

Origin: It originated in Holland and is named after the village of Welsum.

Colors: It is red and black like an old English game bird.

Sizes: It is available in standard and bantam.

Characteristics: These birds have single combs and clean legs. Dark chocolate eggs are produced by those birds that are not such good layers, while lighter brown eggs are produced by hens that lay better.

The eggs are dark brown or light brown and are large. They are friendly birds that love to forage, but they can also adapt to runs. This breed is good for beginners.

White Skinned Chicken Breeds

Andalusians, Blue

Class & Type: These birds are classed as a Mediterranean breed and are a light breed. They are also a very rare breed.

Origin: They originally came from Andalusia, Spain.

Colors: The blue variety is the only one accepted by the APA.

Sizes: Only the standard breed is available

Characteristics: This is a single combed clean legged breed. It is not a brooder and is not known to be docile. It is a good layer of large white **eggs.** It is the original blue chicken, which gave rise to the many blue varieties of chickens. This breed is small and active.

Araucana/Americauna

Class & Type: Araucana/Americauna breeds are classed as "all other breeds."

Origin: Araucunas come from South America. The breed is quite rare they have tufts which make them hard to breed and exhibit.

Colors: The Americauna birds come in Black, Blue Wheaten, Blue, Buff, Wheaten, Brown Red, White and Silver.

Sizes: They come in bantam and standard sizes.

Characteristics: They have beards and muffs but only the Araucunas have tufts. These chickens lay blue colored medium eggs. Aracunas will brood but Americauna breeds will not. They both have pea combs. These birds are breed for their eggs.

Campines

Class & Type: These are a Continental class of breed.

Origin: These birds were developed in Northern Europe.

Colors: Silver and golden are the recognized colors.

Sizes: Standard

Characteristics: This is a single comb clean legged bird. They are not docile birds and are not brooders. They are breed solely for their medium sized white eggs.

Hamburgs

Class & Type: They are classed as a Continental breed.

Origin: They originated in Holland and are an old breed.

Colors: There are a number of colors available Black, White, Silver Penciled, Golden Penciled, Silver Spangled, Golden Spangled,

Sizes: They are a light breed. Bantam as well as standard sizes are available.

Characteristics: They have a rose comb and have clean legs. These birds have a flighty personality and are active which means they need room to forage and are not good in confinement. They lay small white eggs.

Lakenvelders

Class & Type: It is a Continental class breed of chicken and is considered a light breed.

Origin: This breed originated in the Netherlands but was developed in Germany.

Colors: Silver is the color that is accepted for exhibition purposes.

Sizes: Bantam and standard varieties of this breed are available.

Characteristics: It is a good producer of cream or light tinted medium eggs. The breed has a single comb with clean legs. It is not very hardy in winter and it is not a docile bird.

Minorcas

Class & Type: This is a Mediterranean class of breed and is heavier than the other breeds in its class.

Origin: It originated in Spain.

Colors: They are often black with white earlobes. They can be black, white or buff with single combs and white or black with rose combs.

Sizes: They come in bantam and standard sizes.

Characteristics: Is another light breed that lays good sized white eggs. The rooster has a single comb that is large and erect. The hens have a comb that flops over. They can also have rose combs. The chickens do not have a docile disposition and do not brood. They are active and flighty.

Naked Necks

Class & Type: These are classed under all fowl and are a dual purpose bird.

Origin: This breed is Transylvanian but was developed in Germany.

Colors: They come in white, black, red and buff.

Sizes: They come in bantam and standard varieties.

Characteristics: These birds are characterized by their naked neck. They have single combs and clean legs. The birds are docile and friendly. They are fair layers of medium light brown eggs.

White Faced Spanish

Class & Type: One of the oldest breeds this is classed as a Mediterranean breed. It is a medium variety that is bred for eggs.

Origin: It is a Spanish breed.

Colors: Black with a white face and long white earlobes.

Sizes: It comes in standard and bantam varieties.

Characteristics: They have single combs with distinctive white faces and long white earlobes. They are good layers of large white eggs. They are active flighty birds that do not have docile characteristics.

Chapter 5: Dual Purpose Chicken Breeds

How to Raise Chicken for Meat Production

Firstly, you will need to consider the feed to growth ratio and how fast your chickens will grow. Secondly you must not get attached to the chickens, as they must go to slaughter at least 8 weeks. You should choose heavier breeds for meat production and it should have fast growing hybrids.

The birds will need the same requirements as egg laying breeds. These include a clean, dry coop. The birds do not like to roost at night because they are heavier breeds, so you will not need perches. They will need a warm, comfortable place to sleep. You will not need nesting boxes as the birds will be slaughtered before they start to lay.

What Age Should I Start Harvesting?

The birds will be ready for slaughter at around 5 to 8 weeks depending on the rate of growth. You should not slaughter them after 8 weeks or they will become too big and they will have health problems. Older chickens can also get quite tough.

Yellow Skinned Chicken Breeds

Brahmas

Class & Type: This is an Asian class breed and is a heavier breed. It can be used for both eggs and meat.

Origin: India.

Colors: They come in dark, buff and light.

Sizes: The breed comes in standard or bantam.

Characteristics: This breed is a large sized bird and the rooster can grow up to 11 lb. It is feather legged with feathers on its feet and has a pea comb. One rooster is best kept with only two hens. They are good for cold climates. The chickens are docile friendly chickens and are good layers of medium brown eggs.

Buckeyes

Class & Type: This is an American class breed and is considered to be a rare and endangered breed.

Origin: They originated in the state of Ohio in the USA.

Colors: They are dark mahogany.

Sizes: It comes in standard size.

Characteristics: They are a heavy variety of chicken and can be used for both eggs and meat. They have small pea combs and clean legs. It has a quiet disposition.

Chanteclers

Class & Type: They are American class birds and are used for dual purpose.

Origin: These birds originated in Canada.

Colors: The variety comes in partridge and white.

Sizes: They come in bantam and standard sizes.

Characteristics: They are very winter hardy and have small single combs. This breed is a friendly bird and will not brood. Also they lay large brown eggs.

Cochins

Class & Type: This bred is classed as Asian and is a heavy breed used for meat and exhibition purposes.

Origin: These birds originated in China.

Colors: The breed comes in a variety of colors, black, white and lavender.

Sizes: They come in bantam and standard.

Characteristics: These birds have feathered legs and feet and are a heavier breed. They are dual purpose breeds and also used for exhibition purposes. They must be kept on clean flooring that is maintained well so that their feathered legs and feet do not get spoiled. They have small combs that are well-serrated. Their eggs are light brown in color.

Delaware

Class & Type: This is an American class breed, which is a cross between the Plymouth Rock and New Hampshire Reds. It is a heavy breed and quite rare.

Origin: This breed originated in the state of Delaware.

Colors: It is white with black bars on the neck, wing tips and tail.

Sizes: It comes in standard and bantam sizes.

Characteristics: They are very good layers of large brown eggs. They are docile birds and very winter hardy. These chickens will brood. They have single combs and clean legs.

Dominiques

Class & Type: This is an American class chicken and is a dual purpose bird. It is now considered quite rare.

Origin: It had its origins with the Pilgrim Fathers and was probably brought to America by these settlers.

Colors: It is a barred variety of chicken.

Sizes: It comes in standard and bantam.

Characteristics: This breed has a rose comb and lays large brown eggs. It also has clean legs. It is a docile bird and a good brooder.

Hollands

Class & Type: This is an American class of chicken and the breed is now quite rare.

Origin: This breed originated from Holland.

Colors: Barred and white breeds are available.

Sizes: The breed comes in standard and bantam sizes.

Characteristics: This chicken has a single comb with clean legs. They are good brooders and quite friendly birds. They lay large, white eggs and are dual purpose birds.

Javas

Class & Type: This is an American class breed and they are a medium heavy variety.

Origin: They are bred from an unknown Asian breed in the USA.

Colors: The breed comes in white, black and mottled.

Sizes: They come in standard and bantam sizes.

Characteristics: They have single combs and clean legs. The breed is very docile and broods well. It is a dual purpose chicken and can be confined.

Jersey Giants

Class & Type: This is a very heavy breed of chicken that originally was bred for meat. It is classed as an American breed.

Origin: It originated in the US.

Colors: At first only black ones were bred but now Blue laced and White breeds can be seen.

Sizes: It only comes in standard size.

Characteristics: These birds are crosses of Langshans and Brahmas breeds. They are large chickens and can sometimes grow up to 13 pounds. These breeds are bred mainly for meat. The Australorps were also used in the breeding process making some black giants look similar to this breed. They lay brown eggs and can be used for this purpose.

Lamonas

Class & Type: This is an American class of breed and is now considered very rare.

Origin: This breed originated and was developed in the US.

Colors: It comes in white.

Sizes: It was bred as a standard bird but lately there was a bantam breed developed.

Characteristics: It has a single red comb and red earlobes. It lays large white eggs. It is heavier than the White Leghorn but lighter than other meat birds like the Dorking.

New Hampshires

Class & Type: It is an American class of breed

Origin: It originated from the US.

Colors: It is reddish brown.

Sizes: It comes in bantam and standard sizes.

Characteristics: The New Hampshire Red is the most popular of these breeds. This is another breed that is dual purpose; they are also used as exhibition birds. They are easy to breed making them a popular variety for first time flock owners who want to breed their birds. It lays large brown eggs.

Plymount Rocks

Class & Type: This is classed as an American breed. These are dual purpose birds and can be used for meat and eggs.

Origin: It originated from the US.

Colors: It is also known as the Barred Rock due to its black and white barring color.

Sizes: They are a medium breed of chicken that lays brown or cream colored eggs

Characteristics: It has a docile friendly disposition and is ideal for the first time backyard chicken flock. It is an excellent forager.

Wyandottes

Class & Type: It is an American class breed and is a heavier variety.

Origin: This breed originated in America.

Colors: There are several types of this variety. Originally, this breed began as the Silver Laced Wyandotte, now it has at least 22 variations.

Sizes: It is a medium sized bird.

Characteristics: This chicken is another dual purpose one. It is another breed that works well for the beginner. They are docile and good tempered birds.

White Skinned Chicken Breeds

Australorps

Class & Type: This is classed as English breed although it came from Australia.

Origin: This breed originated in Australia.

Colors: It comes in black.

Sizes: This breed comes in standard and bantam.

Characteristics: It is a single comb clean leg breed. It is a dual purpose bird which lays large brown eggs. It is docile and will even sit on eggs. It is a great breed for beginners who want to raise chickens.

Catalanas, Buff

Class & Type: This is a Mediterranean class breed that is bred for its eggs.

Origin: This breed originated in Catalonia, Spain.

Colors: This breed comes in buff.

Sizes: It comes in bantam and standard.

Characteristics: This chicken has clean legs and a single comb. They are not a docile bird and are quite active and flighty by nature. These chickens lay cream colored or slightly tinted eggs. This is a dual purpose chicken.

Crevecoeur

Class & Type: This breed is of the French class and is considered quite rare.

Origin: This breed originated in France.

Colors: It comes in black.

Sizes: This chicken can be found in both bantam and standard sizes.

Characteristics: This breed was bred for meat and is crossed with the Dorking to make it bigger. It also lays a number of white eggs. It has a crest and a V-shaped horned comb. This chicken is susceptible to lice, due to its crest, so it will need to be checked regularly. It is easily tamed making it good for a backyard flock.

Dorkings

Class & Type: This is an English class of breed. It is considered rare.

Origin: It originated in England.

Colors: Red and silver grey varieties should have a single comb. However, the white and cuckoo colors should have a rose comb.

Sizes: It only comes in standard size.

Characteristics: This is an old variety of chicken. It has 5 toes and its body has a boat shape. It is a heavy breed that is bred for meat, egg and exhibition purposes. It is a bird with a pleasant personality.

Faverolles

Class & Type: They are a French class of breed.

Origin: They originally came from France but are now divided into French, British and German breeds.

Colors: The original color is salmon but other countries, apart from the U.S, allow other colors for exhibition. Like white and mahogany.

Sizes: They come in bantam and standard sizes.

Characteristics: This breed is another dual purpose chicken which is good for meat and egg laying production. They have 5 toes, a beard, light feathers on their legs and side muffs.

LaFleche

Class & Type: This breed is considered as a French class of breed and is a heavy variety.

Origin: La Fleche comes from France.

Colors: Originally, they were black chickens but now Blue Laced, Cuckoo and White varieties are available.

Sizes: This breed is available in standard and bantam sizes.

Characteristics: This heavy breed is an old one from France. It has a crest in the shape of 2 horns. The French keep them primarily for meat but they also lay large white eggs.

Langshans

Class & Type: This breed is classed as an Asian breed. This is a dual purpose breed and is considered to be rare.

Origin: It is Chinese in origin.

Colors: It is predominantly black.

Sizes: It comes in bantam and standard sizes.

Characteristics: This breed was developed from a Chinese breed called Croad Langshan. The Croad Langshan was crossbred with Plymouth rocks and Minorcas to improve its egg laying capacity. This cross breed became the Langshan breed. It is known as a heavy bird, with a single 5 pointed comb. It has feathered legs and will lay light brown eggs.

Orpingtons

Class & Type: This breed is classed as an English variety and is a heavy breed.

Origin: It originated in the U.K.

Colors: They come in a number of colors but the most common are buff, blue, white and black

Sizes: Is a heavy breed that also lays well.

Characteristics: The comb is small and single and the chicken is docile and friendly. This makes it a good bird to keep if you are a beginner at chicken raising. It has light brown eggs and is used for both eggs and meat

Redcaps

Class & Type: This breed is classed as English breed.

Origin: This breed originated in England

Colors: They have a red and black plumage; also the hock and saddle feathers of the rooster also have green webbing, which is tipped with black. The hen is nut brown with black half-moon spangles on her feathers.

Sizes: It is a medium heavy breed

Characteristics: This breed is also known as Derbyshire Redcap. It was created as a dual purpose breed, but is now used for its medium, white eggs. It has a large rose comb with a leader that is long and straight.

Rhode Island Reds

Class & Type: This is an American class of breed and is considered to be a medium heavy variety of chicken.

Origin: The United States of America

Colors: The Rhode Island Red is a chestnut brown chicken.

Sizes: It comes in bantam size and standard size.

Characteristics: They are well known for their egg laying prowess and are also heavy enough to be bred for meat. They have a nice disposition and are good for keeping as part of a backyard flock. They will lay good sized brown eggs. They are single combed with clean legs.

Rhode Island Whites

Class & Type: This is classed as an American breed and is classified as a medium heavy breed. The breed is now becoming quite rare.

Origin: The United States of America

Colors: White.

Sizes: Medium heavy

Characteristics: They are a different breed from the Rhode Island

Reds: This breed is a good egg layer of large orange colored eggs and is a large fowl. They have a pleasant disposition but do not get on so well with other breeds. They have a rose comb.

Sussex

Class & Type: This is an English class of breed. They are dual purpose.

Origin: They originated in England.

Colors: It comes in a number of colors but is most well-known for its Columbian plumage with a white body, speckled neck and black tail feathers.

Sizes: They come in bantam and standard sizes.

Characteristics: It has a single comb and the hens are good layers.

Chapter 6: Alternative Chicken Breeds

Some breeds of chicken are quite unusual and can either be kept as pets or for exhibition purposes.

Blue Foot Chicken

Class & Type: This is an American class breed.

Origin: It originated in Canada.

Colors: It comes in white.

Sizes: It comes in standard sizes.

Characteristics: It has a single comb and is characterized by its blue legs. The bird is raised carefully as a delicious meat bird and an exhibition chicken.

Breese Chicken

Class & Type: This is a French class of breed and is bred for meat.

Origin: It originated in France.

Colors: It comes in white.

Sizes: It comes in a standard size.

 Characteristics: It has a single comb and blue legs. It is much prized as a delicious chicken meat.

Houdan

Class & Type: French

Origin: It originated in France.

Colors: There are other colors but the black mottled variety is most common.

Sizes: It comes in standard size only.

Characteristics: This breed was originally bred for meat but is now used for exhibitions, as it is really a light breed of chicken. It is a crested variety and because of this is best kept indoors or in a covered run. Its comb is termed butterfly and it has 5 toes. It requires the same care as Polish breeds due to its crest.

Poulet Rouge Fermier

Class & Type: This is a French class of breed.

Origin: It originated in France.

Colors: It is generally found in light brown.

Sizes: Standard breeds are available.

Characteristics: This breed of chicken was bred for its flavor and is known as one of the best flavored poultry in the world. It is a single small combed chicken and has a naked neck in the US.

Silkie Chicken

Class & Type: This breed is a Feather Legged Bantam class of breed.

Origin: They originated in China.

Colors: They come in Black, Partridge, White, Blue, Buff and Gray.

Sizes: This is a true bantam.

Characteristics: They are good brooders and mothers. Additionally, they make good pets as they are extremely docile. This chicken has 5 toes and a walnut comb with a crest. They are generally kept as pets or for exhibition purposes. This breed comes in bearded and non-bearded varieties.

Sumatras, Black

Class & Type: They are classed as "all other breeds". These chickens are a medium breed of exhibition birds.

Origin: They are related to the original jungle fowl of the Far East.

Colors: Glossy black.

Sizes: This is a medium breed and is available in bantam and standard varieties.

Characteristics: It has a pea comb and although red combed varieties are available, the blue or gypsy combed type is preferred by bird fanciers. They are not very friendly birds and a little wild, but are very beautiful. The roosters can have tails that can grow to 4 feet. They are best kept in free range conditions. Because of their plumage they require higher roosts and dry conditions. They lay medium white eggs but do not lay well.

Chapter 7: Modern Methods of Chicken Production

High Rate of Feed Conversions

This is an important factor when raising chickens especially if they are to be used for meat. It is the amount or pounds of feed the chicken consumes divided by its clean carcass. Most backyard flocks are not very high in feed conversions. This means that they will very likely cost you more to get to the table than commercially bought chickens. Ways to reduce feed is to confine your birds and to get breeds that are fast growing. Different breeds are more feed efficient than others. Cross breeding can sometimes produce more feed efficient birds. If you are raising chickens for meat that will be sold, it is important to buy the right breed of efficient feed to pound ratio.

Rapid Weight Gain

Ideally, your chickens that are bred for meat should have a rapid weight gain and be ready for slaughtering in 5 to 8 weeks. Some breeds will put on more weight than others. The commercial Cornish Cross breed is an example of a breed that will have rapid weight gain. Many chicken farmers will recommend mixing milk or buttermilk in the feed to fatten up chickens. Additionally, table scraps are also good. The chickens should be confined a little so that they take less exercise. Try not to feed them high fiber supplements.

Early Maturity

When raising chickens for meat and eggs, try to select breeds that mature early. These breeds will have a higher rate of feed conversion and be more economical to keep. The New Hampshire breed is known for its early maturity. This is a dual purpose bird that is a good layer and meat bird. Raising chickens for meat or eggs means economical management of feed per bird. Leghorns are excellent layers and are light birds that will consume less feed per bird and will lay at an early age.

Trap Nesting

This is when you will literally trap the chicken as she is laying eggs. This is a method used to check on your laying chickens, whether they have laid eggs and how many eggs they have produced. You can easily see what sort of eggs one chicken has produced and the quality of chicks for breeding purposes. This method will separate your best layers from the rest of the flock.

Culling

It is when you get rid of the birds that you do not need when you are breeding for production of meat and eggs. To get exactly the right breed of bird you will need to cull ruthlessly. When you get too many roosters you also need to sell or slaughter them.

Chapter 8: Proper Ways of Incubating Chicken Eggs

Hatching chicken eggs through incubation requires knowledge and careful planning, if you are going to be successful with your incubation project. To be successful you need to know the best ways to incubate chicken eggs and the solutions to questions that can come up in the process. Here are some answers to basic questions that deal with incubation of chicken eggs so that the result is healthy chickens.

Natural Incubation

The most successful way to incubate chickens is the natural way with a broody hen who sits on her eggs. However, not all breeds are natural mothers and some will not sit on eggs. Two breeds of chickens that are known for being good broody hens are the Brahma breed and the Silkie breed. Chickens either have the instinct to brood or not – it is not something you can force. It is also necessary to have a rooster for fertilization if you want to hatch chicks. As with any form of incubation, not every egg will hatch; there will always be some that fail. The best thing to do for a broody hen is to leave her alone to do her thing as much as possible.

How to Incubate Chicken Eggs

If you decide to artificially incubate chicken eggs with an incubator make sure that the temperature is a steady 99.5 F degrees before you place the eggs in the incubator. It takes roughly 21 days for the eggs to hatch. Humidity also needs to be at 50% for the first eighteen days which will then be increased to 80% in the last few days. Eggs also have to be turned three times a day so use a pencil to mark the eggs so you know which to turn. Put an X on one side and O on the other.

Make Sure the Incubator Temperature is Stable

It is very important that the temperature of the incubator remain stable. To ensure that the incubator is correct it is best to calibrate it before use.

When Should I Increase the Humidity of the Incubator?

Most people who raise chickens think day 19 is the best day to increase the humidity in the incubator to between 65% and 80%. Humidity can be increased by adding wet sponges to the incubator. Some incubators will have a built in humidity regulator.

When Does a Hen Start Sitting on Her Eggs?

Only broody chickens will sit on their eggs for hatching. Most hens have had this trait bred out of them. If they are going to sit on the eggs it will probably be after laying about a dozen eggs.

How Long Does it Take a Hen to Lay Her Eggs?

Hens do not lay eggs until they are at least five months old. Young hens tend to lay one egg approximately every three days. It really depends on the breed.

The Difference between Brown and White Eggs

Nutritionally there is no difference between brown and white eggs; chickens that have white feathers and white ear lobes will lay white eggs while chickens that possess red feathers and lobes lay brown eggs.

What is the Hatching Period of the Chicken Eggs?

Chicken eggs generally take approximately 21-22 days to hatch.

Can a Hen Lay Her Eggs Without a Rooster?

Hens can lay eggs without rooster. It does take a rooster however for the eggs to be fertilized to produce chicks.

Why Do Some Eggs Don't Fertilize?

When roosters mate with hens, sperm is transferred to the oviduct of the hen and then takes up to a week to travel to the infundibulum where it stays for up to a week. If there are yolks present at that time, fertilization will take place. If the conditions are not exactly right an egg will not be fertilized.

How to Make Homemade Incubator

To create a homemade incubator start with a box that measures approximately 2 feet by 2 feet. You want to then cut a hole directly in the middle of the box that will accommodate a light bulb. After putting the light bulb in the hole, add a cup of water in the box, and place fertilized eggs in the box under the bulb. Make sure to check the temperature and humidity and to turn the eggs at least three times daily.

Chicken Nesting Boxes

If you are going to need several nest boxes you can purchase them commercially or you might be able to create them from items you already have. It is possible to create nesting boxes from plastic tubs, wooden crates, 55 gallon drums cut in half, old wash tubs, or a sanitized litter box. The main idea here is to provide a fairly private safe place for nesting. Most experts recommend that a nesting box be provided for no more than three birds. The nesting boxes should be lined with wood shavings or sawdust or similar material.

Wood Nesting Box (Small & Large)

Simple wood nesting boxes are available commercially in feed stores or online in both small and large sizes. A large wood nesting box (20x11x10) will run you approximately $30 and a small nesting box (16x9x10) runs about $15.00.

Chick-n-Nesting Box

The Chick-n-Nesting Box is another inexpensive alternative for egg nesting. These wooden boxes cost about $15.00 and the dimension is approximately 13x11x12.5 inches. Ware is a manufacturer of these boxes.

6-Hole-Chick-Inn Laying Nest

The 6-Hole-Chick-Inn Laying Nest from FarmTek accommodates 24 hens. This multi-level nest box has plastic lids and partitions at the front and the back. The nest is made so that it is easy to keep clean with removable plastic inserts. The nest box is available with individual nest pads. The cost is approximately $170.00.

Ware Premium plus Backyard Hatch

The Ware Premium plus Backyard Hatch is another option. It is a wooden combination pen and hutch which can be used for chickens in addition to rabbits, guinea pigs, ferrets, and other small animals. It retails for between $70 – and $150.00.

How to Make a Simple Chicken Nest Box

It is possible to construct a slanted nest box with a front opening for a chicken. Broody chickens look for quiet dark locations to nest and you can create the perfect nest box to interest them. You will need a saw, drill, two 1x12x 16 ½" which you are going to cut at a slant of 20% off square on one side (2 sides), 1 1x12x12 (bottom), 2 1x2x12 (top supports), 4 5 ½" fence pickets at 13 ½" long (back and one front piece), and 3 5 ½" fence pickets at 15 ½" long (roof). Note: You do not have to use pickets if you can use a solid piece of wood for the top of the slanted box instead. Start with assembling the base and the two sides, and then add the top supports flush to the inside with screws and wood glue. Then attach the four pickets to create the solid back and the front piece. Finish up with the remaining pickets for the roof slanted with a 1" overhang and the pieces stacked one in front of the other (partially covering the other piece).

Different Type of Incubators

There are lots of choices when it comes to incubators. Choose an incubator based on the specific requirements for use. There are commercial sized incubators, homemade incubators and everything in between. You can find incubators that come with heating elements, fans, humidity controls, flexible egg trays, and automatic egg turning. Prices start at $20 and go up. Different types of incubators include educational incubators used in schools or 4-H, hobby farm incubators, and large commercial incubators.

Basic Incubator

You can make your own incubator or purchase a basic type of egg incubator. You can purchase fairly simple incubators that come with an automatic egg turner, a digital thermometer, and a hygrometer to measure humidity so that you have everything you need. Check out the Little Giant Basic Incubator Combo Kit which runs about $95.00.

Cabinet Incubator

Cabinet incubators are great for people who are seriously into hatching large numbers of chicken eggs. They can also be used for other types of fowl eggs. The larger cabinet incubators come with a digital thermostat with LCD constant displays for both temperature and humidity. Some models even come with computer monitor systems so that you can keep an eye on egg rotation, and audio and visual indicators. Egg capacity for a cabinet incubator can accommodate almost 300 chicken eggs or more.

Precision Incubator

Precision incubators are good for commercial use as some models can hold more than 5,000 chicken eggs at a time. Precision incubators are fully automatic and most of them are energy efficient.

Industrial-Sized Incubator

Industrial size incubators are generally completely computerized and automated and can incubate more than 100,000 eggs in a controlled environment in terms of temperature, humidity, ventilation and egg turning.

Homemade Incubator

If you are just getting started with raising chickens from eggs you can start out cheaply with a homemade incubator constructed from cardboard boxes, plywood or a Styrofoam ice chest. You will need to determine if the incubator will be a still air incubator or moving air incubator with the addition of a fan.

Chicken Eggs Hatch Rate

Average of Broodiness Hen

Broody hens will depend on the breed. Generally the egg laying breeds like the Leghorn and other Mediterranean breed bred for egg laying are more skittish and will not brood. However the heavier breeds that are dual purpose birds are more inclined to breed and be good mothers. Examples of good brooders are the Silkie in the bantam class and New Hampshire in standard breeds.

Cost: It will cost $0 to hatch and raise chicks naturally as the mother hen will hatch the eggs herself and look after the chicks.

Homemade Incubator

You will need a 2 ft by 2ft square box and you will make a circular hole in the top. In this hole you will insert your heat lamp. A cup of water should be placed in the box for humidity. Fertilized eggs will then be placed under the heat lamp. The eggs will need to be turned x2 or x3 per day. The humidity should be kept at 60 degrees to 65 degrees and the temperature should be about 99 degrees. After the first 18 days leave the eggs alone and be sure that the eggs are not disturbed.

Cost

The box can be an old cooler and if it is just lying around will cost you nothing.

The heat lamp kit should cost around $6.00

A thermometer which tells you how warm it is in the incubator would cost around $1.00

A piece of glass to fit on the roof or lid of the thermos, this will be under a dollar.

You may want to have something to measure humidity, which will not cost more than $5.00

The whole project could be done below $20.00

If you get the eggs from your own chickens then it will be of no additional cost.

Industrial Incubator or Artificial Incubator

An industrial or artificial incubator will take quite a number of eggs. It will have automatic temperature and humidity gages so that you do not have to worry about this. Observation windows will be available for looking at the hatching process. The more expensive ones will have automatic egg turners.

Cost:

The incubator, without automatic egg turner will cost around $60 and about $130 with automatic egg turner. The entire cost for the project will be around $150. Again you can use eggs from your own chickens to cut costs.

Chapter 9: Tips for the Newbies Chicken Breeder

The goals of poultry farming

Going into poultry farming either as a hobby or as a business means that you have decisions to make about whether you are going to be primarily in the egg production business or the hatchery business or other facets of the poultry farming industry. Some individuals go into poultry farming simply because they want to have fresh eggs available that they know come from a healthy clean environment. Others are interested in raising chicks to sell. No matter what the goal is if you are going to be in the poultry farming business you will need to know all the different aspects of taking care of chickens.

Making a budget plan

It is important to make a budget plan for any venture such as raising chickens either as a backyard venture or as a commercial business. The amount of the budget and capital depends on the size of the venture. Even a backyard poultry business will require a minimum of several hundred dollars up to $10,000 depending on the size of the flock and the size of the business. Estimate veterinarian care into your expenses which can run up to $100 plus per visit. Breeding chickens to sell either fertile eggs or day old chicks can be lucrative but does require time, planning and investment.

Feed expense

The cost of feeding chickens is relative to the size of the flock. It is estimated that to feed four chickens it will cost approximately $20.00 per month in chicken feed. Supplemental vitamins and other products will increase the cost. If you are operating a backyard type poultry farm you can use clean household food scraps as part of the feed. An adult six pound hen will eat approximately three pounds of chicken feed per week.

Water systems

It is essential that chickens have fresh clean water available to them at all times. With young chicks especially the water needs to be from a device that prevents drowning. There are a variety of different watering devices and systems to accommodate different budgets and types of poultry businesses. Commercial systems use circulating water systems with a filter.

Waste management

Chicken areas and coops must be kept clean of chicken manure. An average chicken around four pounds produce on average a .0035 cubic feet of manure each day. It is recommended that chicken coops be cleaned once a week or twice a week. Chicken manure can be used in compost piles though to keep odor and flies down. The moisture level should be reduced to eliminate problems.

Proper farm locations

The right location for your poultry farm depends on the size of your business, local zoning laws, and whether your chickens will be free ranging or kept in a coop or run. If you will be operating a commercial venture you will want to have enough land to run the business without causing odor problems or noise for other residents. You will also want to consider whether the business is close to a feed store or will feed be delivered and it is important to identify where your customers are located.

Invest with the best breed of chickens

One of the first things to consider when starting your poultry business is what poultry breeds you will be raising. There are breeds that are better for egg production, and backyard businesses. Popular breeds include the Rhode Island Red, the Wayndotte, the Ameraucana and the Orpington. Check with other local chicken farmers or breeder to see which breeds do the best in your area.

Find a trusted chicken supplier

Finding the right supplier for your flock is probably the most important decision you will make in starting your poultry farm. A good place to begin your search for a reputable breeder is your local agricultural State University Cooperative Extension Service. They can often provide information on local poultry farming. Ask other poultry farmers for recommendations and check references on the business. Some large commercial outfits that ship live chicks send baby roosters as packing material to keep the female chicks warm. Chicks that are shipped through the mail will be without food or water for several days and can be exposed to extreme temperatures.

Know what breed you are hatching

One way to find a good supplier if you are ordering live chicks or hatching fertilized eggs is to ask whether the supplier will be able to ensure that you will receive the exact breed that you want. Suppliers who ship fertilized eggs should provide breed codes with each shipment.

Don't buy mixed breed hatching eggs

Not all poultry breeders agree with the premise that you should not breed chickens from mixed breed eggs. However some breeders believe that mixed breed eggs can be problematic and in some cases not viable.

Avoid overcrowding chickens

The more space you can provide chickens the happier they will be. Chickens that are kept in small coops are likely to be exposed to unhealthy levels of manure and are more likely to peck at each other. For large birds, each bird should have a minimum of four square feet while smaller birds require a minimum of two square feet.

Don't touch the first born chicks

It is better not to handle first born chicks. Day old chicks can be handled but you want to be sure that you are doing so with gloves or very clean hands so that you don't introduce germs. In addition, always wash your hands after handling chicks to protect yourself from their germs. If you will be raising the chickens as pets you will want to get them used to being handled but keep young children from over handling young chicks.

Always monitor the growth of your chicks

From the minute you have your chicks they should be monitored in terms of their health, the temperature and cleanliness of their environment and access to clean water and food.

When should I move the chicks into a brooder?

Day old chicks can be moved directly into a heated brooder or the chicks' first home. Some breeders move new hatchlings after two hours in the incubator. It is important to remember that if there are chicks still hatching opening the incubator can cause a loss of required humidity which could lead to loss of chicks.

Place them in a well-ventilated coop

Whatever type of shelter you provide for your flock you want to make sure that it is well ventilated without being drafty. In hot months there should be free air movement through the coop and in winter months it is essential to keep the chickens warm. Coops also need to be predator proof.

How long should I light my chicks with incandescent bulb? How many watts are recommended?

If you are going to be using a light bulb as a heat source then you will need a variety of standard light bulbs in 100 watt, 75 watt, 60 watt and a 40, and a 25 watt bulb. At first the chicks will need the 100 watt bulb for the first week, and then you can go down to the 75 for week two, 60 watt for week three and 40 watt for fourth week. A 25 watt bulb will work fine after the first month.

Proper handling of the eggs

It is important that all eggs from your flock that you will be using for food be handled safely. Salmonella and other bacteria can be found on the shell. Nest boxes need to be kept clean and eggs should be gathered at least once a day. Eggs can be cleaned with rinsing with a spray bottle of warm water and then wiped with a paper towel. Make sure to wash your hands thoroughly before and after handling eggs. Store all eggs with the larger ends facing up at 50-55 degrees. If you are preserving fertilized eggs for sale you will want to keep them at a 55 degree temperature and you will have to turn the eggs daily until they are placed in an incubator. The sooner they are place in an incubator the better – they will remain hatchable for approximately five to seven days.

Give them vaccine

There is controversy over whether to vaccinate poultry. However veterinarians recommend that poultry be vaccinated due to the number of severe diseases that can affect chickens such as Marek's Disease a particularly virulent and deadly disease.

Keep everything clean

One way to prevent disease is by adhering to strict guidelines for cleanliness with the flock. It is essential that the coops and surrounding areas be kept clean and there should always be clean water available for the chickens.

Maintain health

By keeping coop areas clean and providing enough space, ventilation and fresh water for the chickens you are going a long way in helping to maintain the health of the flock. Keep a vigilant eye on the flock so that if one is showing signs of illness it can be taken care of right away. As a precaution do not bring new chickens into an established flock right away. Any new chicks or chickens should be isolated for a few weeks to ensure healthiness.

Protect them from bad weather

Chickens are affected by weather extremes of cold or hot weather and rain. The living conditions for chickens should provide basic care at all times including reasonable temperatures, dry conditions, and free from draught or high winds. If your chickens have a pen area and you live in an area where there is a lot of snow or rain, provide a tarp or covered area for the flock.

Maintain a regular check-up

If you are running a poultry business whether it is commercial or just a backyard operation, you have made an investment in your poultry and in their health. It is a good idea to have them checked over on a regular basis to ensure good health.

Consult a Veterinarian

You will find it is necessary to use veterinary care for your chickens. Just like any other animal, chickens can get sick and they can get hurt. Be sure to find a veterinarian that is familiar with poultry in your area.

Vaccinate Your Chicks

Most new chicks in commercial enterprises are immediately vaccinated for Marek's disease. Vaccine tends to come in large containers which can be a problem for small backyard farmers. If you are getting your chicks from a commercial outfit check to see if they will be vaccinated before you purchase them.

Separate Diseased Chicken

At the first sign of illness in a bird, isolate them from the rest of the flock. Signs of illness in a chicken can include difficulty breathing, coughing or wheezing, feather loss, fever, a wound, stiffness, discharge or diarrhea, and not eating or drinking.

Disposing of Dead Chicks or Chicken Properly

There can be a high mortality rate for chicks. Chickens are more likely to die from predators but they also can become sick with disease. Disposing of dead birds needs to be done in accordance with local health laws. In most areas, acceptable disposal methods include composting and incineration. Depending on the size of the poultry business, you must have a disposal system in place.

Chapter 10: Building Your Chicken Coop

What are the Criteria of Building a Chicken Coop?

A chicken coop should meet the minimum needs and basic care requirements for your chicken flock. Basic requirements include providing enough space for your chickens that is comfortable, meets safety requirements in terms of keeping predators out, dry, ventilated but not drafty and easy to clean.

What are the Tools and Materials to Build a Chicken Coop?

Tools and materials that you will need to build a chicken coop depend on the style of coop you will be building. There are lots of different types of chicken coops from mobile to stationary to one floor to multiple floors and they can be made out of wood, metal or plastic. However, basic building equipment is likely to require some basic tools such as a hammer, circular saw, tape measure, safety equipment, drill, level, square, wire cutters or tin snips, and possibly a screw gun.

How to Build a Mobile Chicken Coop

A mobile chicken coop is exactly what it sounds like in that the coop can be moved around. If you have the land for chickens to free range, a mobile chicken coop can be moved when needed providing shelter and protection from predators. To build a mobile chicken coop you can use wood or something lighter. To create your mobile chicken coop you can repurpose small sheds or even a dog house or a stationary chicken coop and then make it mobile by adding wheels. Mobile chicken coops can also be created without wheels but are light enough and easy enough to dismantle and move. For inspiration you can find a variety of plans at sites such as Mother Earth News, and College Agricultural Extension divisions.

How to Clean a Chicken Coop

Keeping a chicken coop clean is how you help ensure that your flock stays healthy. Most people depending on the size of the flock and the chicken coop do a full cleaning every one to two weeks. The chickens need to be removed from the coop first. Using gloves, remove the shavings. Some clean the floor using a special coop cleaner or a water and vinegar mixture. At this point, you may want to spray the walls and all other areas with a poultry protector which can help prevent infestation with mites and lice. Replace the pine shavings or whatever you are using on the floor.

Steps for sanitizing the coop

- Regularly clean the chicken poop everyday.

- Do a complete clean and sanitization as described above once a week. This will include putting clean bedding in the nesting boxes and scrubbing down the roosts.

- Clean, fresh feed and water must be provided to the chickens on a daily basis.

For Sale Chicken Coop

There are a variety of different types of chicken coops that are reasonable in cost that you can purchase from feed companies, or online. For a small backyard flock chicken coops made from wood and other materials with screened in areas and runs are available starting at about $70.00 and upwards.

Chicken Fencing

You will want to use some type of fencing around your coop or chicken area to protect your flock from predators and to keep out rodents and other pests. Some popular types of fencing include galvanized hardware cloth, chicken wire, chain link, rabbit wire, and electric net fencing. Chicken wire is probably the least effective at keeping predators out.

DIY chicken house

One of the easiest and cheapest ways to construct a chicken coop or chicken house is to purchase a Do It Yourself kit. They tend to be easy to put together and inexpensive. E-Z Frames offers a variety of kits starting at about $70.00. The wire structures can then be partially covered in roofing material to provide the chickens with shade. There are also wooden chicken house kits available at different price points that are more substantial including both stationary and mobile coops.

Renovating a Chicken Coop

Another relatively inexpensive way to create or change a chicken coop is to renovate a used one or alter the one you already have. Reasons for altering an existing coop could be to add more ventilation, provide more space for health reasons, or increase the size of a run to add more area for chickens to exercise. You may also want to renovate an existing coop to make it mobile. The budget for renovating a coop will depend on how extensive your renovations will be. Be sure to look at the costs between renovating and purchasing or building a new structure before you begin with your renovation.

Portable Chicken Tractor

A portable chicken tractor generally refers to the type of chicken coop that does not have a floor so chickens have access to grass and other forage. Common types of portable chicken tractors are A-frame coops which are sometimes called arks.

A chicken tractor is another name for a mobile chicken coop. Generally they do not have floors and can be moved around a yard at will. It can save on cleaning a coop but can be problematic in bad weather.

Stationary Chicken Coop

Stationary chicken coops are probably the most popular types of chicken coops though experienced poultry farmers will tell you that portable chicken coops make for happier chickens. One of the advantages of a stationary chicken coop particularly if you are backyard farmer is that you can make the chicken coop look homey and make it fit into the landscape.

Wooden Chicken Coop

Chicken coops made out of wood are available in both portable and permanent structures. You can build your own or use a kit or a plan to create a wooden chicken coop. Most wooden structures will include nest boxes, and perches for birds to sleep and open areas for ventilation.

Plastic Chicken Coop

For the latest in convenience, there are also plastic chicken coops such as the popular Eglu from Omlet Ltd in the UK. This unit is for small scale poultry farming and is an award winning design. It measures 120x60x48 and weighs approximately 43 pounds. Another model is the Snap Lock Chicken Coop which is an easy to assemble coop constructed of light weight plastic that does not require maintenance.

Pre-Made Chicken Coop

If you are looking for a readymade chicken coop with little or no assembly you have lots of models to choose from. You can find inexpensive backyard hutches to kits that require only simple assembly that will house a fairly large number of chickens.

Small Chicken Coop

With the growing popularity of having backyard poultry farms, there are thousands of small chicken coops that you can buy or plans you can use to create a small chicken coop. They are available from local feed stores or from farm websites and you will even find that on sites such as amazon.com.

Medium Chicken Coop

A medium size backyard chicken coop will comfortably house approximately four hens or six bantams depending on which medium model you choose. One of the most popular types of medium size coops are the wooden ark design that has been used in the UK for many years.

Large Chicken Coop

A good size large chicken coop for a poultry farmer looking to house about 40 birds would be approximately 10x10. For a large chicken coup look for one that comes with nesting boxes, windows, good ventilation, and enough area for you to move around in for cleaning.

Chicken Coop from Scratch

Building your own chicken coop from scratch is an increasingly popular DIY project to do. There are thousands of free plans for chicken coops in books and online. Base your design on your specific needs for the size of your flock and the area you have for your chickens.

Chicken Brooder

Once your chicks are ready to move from an incubator you will want to move them to a brooder house. Brooders can be created from cardboard boxes to thermostatically regulated ready to use housing.

Chapter 11: Chicken Nutri Feeds and Feeding Chickens

Different Chicken Feeds

Chick Starter

You usually feed the chicks this chick starter until they are about 6 weeks old. Egg/meat chickens will have broiler feed which will make them grow fast. Some farmers will feed their flock on chicken scratch until they are ready to lay at about 4 to 6 months. They will then feed them lay mash or pellets.

Chicken Scratch

This is a mix of whole grains like, oats, wheat rye and corn. The corn or maize should be cracked before mixing in scratch feed. In commercial brands, there will be more corn and maize in the mix. You can make your own blend and keep it in the fridge to keep it fresh. It will last up to a month.

Greens

These are leafy vegetables like spinach, kale and lettuce. They should be cut up and fed to the chickens daily. They will provide lots of vitamins and minerals, including calcium which is very important for laying hens.

Soybeans

This will provide extra protein for the chickens. It is good for all layers and meat birds.

Pellets

Pellets can be fed to the birds when they are 8 weeks and over. A mother bird will break these up for the small chickens but you can start by breaking them up in the first week.

Layer Mash

Instead of pellets some farmers like to give laying birds this ground up type of feed. This layer feed will have more calcium for stronger shells in hens that are bred for laying. It will also have added protein.

Premix

This is a mix of all the vitamins, minerals, medications and nutrients that a chicken will need. They are made for chicks, layers and broilers. This feed has everything mixed in it.

Fish Meal

This is used as a supplement for chicken feed. It is full of protein and Omega 3 and also has minerals and vitamins. Fish meal is all natural and boosts the immune system of the chickens.

Whole Grains

These are mixed together as scratch feed. They are whole grains like oats, wheat and corn, which are not ground.

Steps to Feeding Your Chickens

Give Enough Food and Water at all Times

You should always give fresh food and water to your chickens. Bear in mind that they are birds and will peck and search for eatables all day. They do forage if given the chance but they should have feeds available to them. The best way to feed them is to give them a container of feeds so that they can just help themselves to. A container of feeds placed in a shady spot of the run will satisfy their needs. Cool water should also be placed in a shady part of the run and be available at all times. The feeds and water should be changed daily.

Keep Feeds Stored in Cool and Dry Place

Feed should be kept in a cool dry place. Closed metal containers are good so that vermin like rats and mice do not get into the feed.

Avoid Expired Feeds

Do not get too much feed at a time and always check the expiry date. Wet or moldy feed will make your birds sick and they can even die. To avoid this problem always make sure that your feed is fresh and within the expiry date. Homemade feeds can last about a month in refrigerated conditions.

Grits Should Be Limited to Ensure Proper Digestion

Grit is an important part of a bird's digestive process. They do not have teeth so their gizzards will grind down the hard shells in their diet with the aid of grit.

There are 2 sorts of grit insoluble and soluble. Soluble grit will be broken down by the stomach acid in the bird's digestive system. It is not that effective for grinding food down, but is a good source of calcium. Examples of this are cuttlebone and ground up oyster shells. Insoluble grit is made up of small stones, sand and gravel and will act as teeth for the bird by grinding up hard portions of their diet like seed shells.

However pet birds including chickens do not eat as many hard shelled seeds as domestic birds. Therefore the need for insoluble grit is not so necessary. Foraging chickens will pick up small grains of sand and little stones instinctively. This will be enough to help them with their digestion. Chickens in a closed run require a small amount of grit in their diet. Do not place a dish of grits in the run with the birds as they can overindulge on grits and it will accumulate in the gizzard, causing impaction. A better idea is to mix a small amount with their feed to help their digestion.

Chapter 12: Chicken Diseases

4 Main Types of Chicken Diseases

Metabolic Disease

These are diseases that affect the chicken's metabolic system. The causes of these diseases can be genetic or hereditary. Factors that can cause problems are also poor nutrition or not getting enough feed. Sometimes the chicken is unable to absorb the nutrients from its food. Examples of these metabolic diseases are Cage Layer Fatigue, Rickets and Fatty Liver Syndrome.

Nutritional Disease

These diseases are tied in with metabolic diseases and cause by inadequate nutrients from the chicken's diet. They can have a high mortality rate.

Infectious Disease

There are many diseases that can infect your chickens. Infectious diseases are caused by a variety of pathogens. They can infect the chickens through water, food or air. They are usually very contagious and can easily be carried from bird to bird. Examples of these diseases are Salmonellas, Newcastle Disease and Fowl Pox.

Infections can be devastating to your flock and some diseases require destroying infected birds. Isolation of sick birds is a must and daily checking of your chickens is important. Many infectious diseases are due to poor hygiene and dirty food and water. It is a good preventive measure to keep the coop, feed and water utensils clean. A covered run is also good as many diseases are carried by wild birds.

Parasitic Disease

These diseases are caused by parasites using your chickens as hosts. They can be contracted from another infested chicken. These parasites can also live in cracks in the coop or bedding and come out at night to feast on your chickens while they are sleeping. Examples of these are Parasitic Worms, Lice and Mites.

Common Chicken Diseases, Causes, Symptoms and Their Treatment

Fatty Syndrome

Symptoms: This disease occurs when an abnormal amount of fat cells are deposited in the liver of the bird. It is a serious disease that can result in death if not treated.

Some chickens will show very few symptoms and will just die. Initially signs of the disease are lethargy, depression and loss of appetite. An enlarged liver can be felt due to the fat deposits and the chicken will display a distended abdomen. Egg laying will decrease dramatically and poor feather growth may be observed. Advanced symptoms can include Central Nervous System problems.

Causes: There are a variety of causes for this disease and the actual cause of it is not really known. It can be due to high fat content in the diet, which can occur if the birds have a diet consisting of only seeds, and overeating can also cause this. Disorders such as diabetes and thyroid issues can give rise to this problem. Nutritional deficiencies and hereditary problems are also factors. Toxins in the air, water or feed can also precipitate this disease.

Treatment: The diet for these birds should be low in fat and be high quality pellets. They should also be given plenty of green leafy vegetables and fresh water. Because the birds may be disinclined to eat you may have to feed them through a tube. They need a little extra heat and if in advanced stages may need lactose medicine.

Avian Influenza

Symptoms: This is a disease that is carried by a virus and there are 15 strains of it. The Asiatic strain is the most dangerous as this can infect humans. There will be a dramatic drop in egg laying. The bird will show signs of listlessness and be sitting quietly instead of showing activity that is common to chickens. They may also display runny stool and a cough. They can also show signs of difficulty in breathing and excretions from their nose region.

Causes: This disease is very contagious and can quickly spread from contaminated birds. Wild birds are carriers and can infect chickens if they have contact with the chicken's food and water. It is carried in the feces of the birds.

Treatment: It is good to have a covered run to prevent chickens having contact with wild birds. If birds are seen with these symptoms, they should be isolated quickly and all surfaces that they have been in contact with disinfected promptly. Birds that have the disease are often culled promptly. Vaccinations are sometimes given for some strains.

Avian Encephalomyelitis

Symptoms: This disease causes a dramatic drop in egg production. If chicks under 3 weeks contract it they can have neurological problems. Lack of co-ordination and tremors can be observed in chickens. 25%to

60% of the infected birds die. Chicks will experience weakness, inactivity and sometimes blindness.

Causes: This can be caused by hereditary infection from the mother to chicks and from infected birds. It is a virus.

Treatment: Vaccination or eye drops can be administered to the flock.

Cage Layer Disease

Symptoms: This disease affects young birds that are in the prime of their egg laying capabilities. They display fragile bones and an inability to stand. The birds will stop eating and their egg shells will become thin.

Causes: This problem usually affects battery hens. It is caused by extreme calcium deficiency.

Treatment: Supplementary feedings of calcium and multivitamins will help. It will also help the condition if fewer birds are kept in the space. Good nutrition and availability of fresh water can also help.

Chicken Pox: (Fowl Pox)

Symptoms: Symptoms of this disease are many lesions on parts of the skin that are not feathered. Lesions around the eyes may cause closure of the eye and lesions found around the nostrils may result in a runny nose. As the disease progresses, the lesions will form on the digestive tract and respiratory system. If the disease becomes systemic then lesions can be seen on internal organs. The death rate is moderate; unless it is systemic then you will have more deaths.

Causes: The disease can be spread by mosquitoes and the crusts from lesions of infected birds. It is a virus infection.

Treatment: Vaccination in the first weeks of life and at between 12 and 16 weeks. The chickens should develop a scab or liaison at the vaccination site. If the birds are kept warm and dry and given soft food to eat they can recover. Keep sick birds and their feed and water containers separately, also always wash hands after handling them.

Botulism

Symptoms: Tremors will occur and paralysis. Death is quick.

Causes: Contaminated food and water.

Treatment: There is no vaccine but you can treat sick birds with Epsom salts dissolved in 1 ounce of warm water. The bird should have this several times a day. Food and water should be changed every day and the contamination can be cleaned with disinfectant.

Fowl Cholera

Symptoms: This disease affects birds over 4 months. They have swollen joints with green or yellowish colored diarrhea.

Causes: Wild birds, raccoons and rats carry this disease. It can be carried on contaminated shoes and clothing.

Treatment: It is fatal and any bird that contracts it should be killed as they will become a carrier. Take care of contaminated clothes and shoes and have a covered run to keep wild birds and animals out.

Infectious Bronchitis

Symptoms: The chicken will be wheezing, sneezing and have watery excretion from nose and eyes.

Causes: It is a viral disease.

Treatment: It is very contagious and will result in 50% death rate in chicks. Vaccine should be given to the chickens when they are 15 weeks. The hens will stop egg-laying.

Infectious Coryza

Symptoms: Chickens will have swollen heads, wattles and combs. The eyes can be so swollen that they are shut and sticky discharge is oozing from eyes and nose.

Causes: Other contaminated birds, surfaces and the air.

Treatment: The birds will need to be destroyed.

Marek's Disease

Symptoms: Chickens under 20 weeks are infected. Tumors both externally and internally are present. Paralysis is also seen plus irises of the eyes will turn grey.

Causes: This is a highly contagious disease. It is spread by a virus and becomes airborne from the feather follicles of infected birds.

Treatment: The chicks are vaccinated at 1 day old. If they are infected, they are usually destroyed as they can become carriers.

MoniLiasis (Thrush)

Symptoms: A white cheesy looking growth will appear around their crop. Their appetite will be increased and laying capacity will be decreased. The chicken's feathers will be ruffled and droopy in appearance.

Causes: If chickens eat moldy feed or contaminated water they can get this problem. Sometimes if they have been on antibiotics it can cause this ailment.

Treatment: There is no vaccine for this problem. The condition is usually treated with Nystatin, which can be obtained from the vet. Water and food containers must be disinfected and fresh water and feed should be provided daily.

Mycoplasmosis/CRD/Air Sac Disease

Symptoms: Egg-laying will be decreased and initially weakness in the chicken can be observed. Signs of acute infection can be swollen joints and trouble in breathing. Wheezing sneezing and coughing can be present.

Causes: Wild birds may carry the disease. The mother hen can transmit the infection to the chick through the egg if she has the disease.

Treatment: Vaccines are available and a course of antibiotics may be recommended by the vet.

Newcastle Disease

Symptoms: Wheezing and difficulties in breathing will be present. Paralysis of the legs and wings are present and the eyes appear cloudy. The neck is twisted

Causes: Wild birds can contaminate the chickens and surfaces, or birds with the disease can pass it on to other chickens.

Treatment: Vaccines are available. There is a high mortality of birds that contract the disease below 6 months.

Chicken Anemia Virus

Symptoms: Anemia, lethargy hemorrhage, a decrease in appetite and depression can be seen. It is apparent in young birds and chicks and can lead to death.

Causes: It can be caught from other birds in the flock and transferred through the egg or semen with breeding birds.

Treatment: As chicks get older, they will develop immunity to the disease. Vaccination of breeders before they start laying eggs is recommended. There is no vaccination of broiler chickens.

Omphalitis

Symptoms: This affects the navel of the chicken. It can appear inflamed and will sometimes have a scab. There will be a wet spot on the abdomen and the navel will not heal normally. There will often be multiple infections present and 15% mortality in the chickens. The chicks will be disinclined to eat and drink and will often be dehydrated. They will huddle under the lamp and be depressed. The chicks will not absorb the yolk of the egg.

Causes: Unhygienic conditions in the incubator or incorrect temperature and humidity can give rise to this problem.

Treatment: Keep everything clean and check the temperature and humidity of the incubator. Remember to clean the incubator between hatches. There are no medications for this.

Pullorum

Symptoms: Egg-laying will be decreased and the chicken will sneeze and cough.

Causes: It is a contagious disease and can be passed on to other birds very easily. Wild birds, rodents, insects and even people can carry this disease.

Treatment: There is no treatment for this disease and the infected birds must be destroyed as they will be carriers of the disease, even if they recover.

Pasting

Symptoms: This is usually found in chicks and should be checked for everyday for the first week or so. It is when feces gets stuck around the vent and can cause blockage and death in the chick.

Causes: Stress or over handling can produce this problem.

Treatment: Clean the area well, with a warm washcloth.

Rickets

Symptoms: The disease causes weakness of the bones. The chicks will not be able to walk properly and in severe cases will not be able to breathe. The chick's beaks will be soft.

Causes: This is caused by nutritional deficiencies of Vitamin D3, Phosphorus and calcium. With carefully balanced commercial feeds, this problem does not usually occur. When using homemade recipes be sure to make the feed properly balanced nutritionally.

Treatment: Using properly balanced feeds will eliminate the problem and cure any deficiencies that the chicks may have. Use supplements 3 times the recommended dose of Vitamin D3.

Brooder Pneumonia

Symptoms: The birds breathe with difficulty and have white diarrhea.

Causes: This is a fungal infection and can infect birds through wet, rotten wood in the coop. Moldy feed can also cause this problem.

Treatment: The brooder should be kept warm and dry. Fresh feed and water should be given daily and the food should be kept in airtight dry and cool containers. The brooder should be cleaned regularly.

Coccidiosis

Symptoms: This is a parasite that gets into the chicken's gut. The first signs will be blood in the stool. Egg production will decrease and the birds will be lethargic.

Causes: The parasite can be found in dirty water, damp living conditions and the stool of infected birds.

Treatment: Coxiod can be added to the drinking water of the chickens. Giving the birds vinegar-garlic solution can help to prevent outbreaks. The chicks should be vaccinated against this parasite. Coxiod can be added to their drinking water to prevent infection.

Salmonella

Symptoms: This is a bacterium that lives in the gut of many animals including chickens. There are often no symptoms but if the birds get sick they can exhibit purple colored wattles and combs. They will be lethargic. They will also have a decreased appetite and increased water consumption. Egg-laying will be decreased.

Causes: Rat and rodent droppings in the feed and contamination from other birds. Sometimes chicks can get sick because they are born with the disease that is passed on from their mothers.

Treatment: Keep your chickens clean and clean their housing regularly. Check them regularly for any symptoms of the disease. Sometimes chicks can come with the disease so try to purchase chicks from a reputed hatchery.

Cryptosporidiosis

Symptoms: Sometimes there are few symptoms but chickens can have chronic digestive and respiratory problems. They can exhibit swollen eyes, difficulty in breathing, wheezing and sneezing. They can also have ruffled feathers and diarrhea.

Causes: This is a parasite that can infect other chickens from sick birds' droppings or contaminated shoes and clothing.

Treatment: Sick birds should be isolated and good sanitization observed.

Lice and Mites

Symptoms: You will find these parasites either on your birds or hiding in the cracks of the coop. The birds can be weak and show lethargy. They will become weak and can even die if heavily infected.

Causes: They can be picked up from wild birds and bird shows.

Treatment: Routine checking of the birds and cleaning of the coop is required. You need be especially careful of crested varieties of chickens as lice can hide in their crests. You will need to dust the infected birds.

Toxoplasmosis

Symptoms: Weight loss and decrease in appetite will be seen. A shrunken comb and lack of coordination. Diarrhea is also present and the chicken can go blind.

Causes: A parasite is responsible for this. Wild and domestic cats can be carriers and this disease can be contracted through infected feces.

Treatment: Good hygiene and cleaning are important. Other pets should be kept away from chickens. When disinfecting the coop try not to house any chickens there for 4 weeks.

Behavioral Disease

There are a number of behavioral diseases of chickens. Many of these are due to stress and cramped living conditions.

Symptoms: Chickens will display signs of pecking at each other and will sometimes start an egg eating habit.

Causes: Stress factors include cramped living conditions, too much light in the coop and less food and water.

Treatment: Give plenty of room to the chickens and do not leave the light on in the coop longer than 10 hours for winter laying. Allowing your backyard flock to free range will keep them happy and stress free. Egg eating must be stopped before it becomes a habit. Sometimes it is due to lack of calcium or too much stress.

Chapter 13: How to Keep Chickens Free from Disease

Feeding Management

In order to keep the chickens healthy, it is important to keep their food and water clean. They are birds and as such are not particularly clean. They will pass poop anywhere including around the food and water utensils. Therefore it is very important to change water and give fresh food daily.

Chicken Coop Management

To prevent disease the chicken coop must be kept clean. It is wise to clean it daily and then do a detailed clean up once a week. All natural cleaners like lemon juice for disinfecting the walls are good. This will keep the chickens in good health and they will not suffer from ill effects of chemicals. Nesting boxes and roosts are necessary for the chickens especially if they are egg layers.

Health Management

Aside from keeping the coop clean, the chickens should be kept as stress free as possible. Some flock owners put herbs in the nesting boxes. You should always give the chickens adequate room. Each standard bird needs about 4 feet square. The best way to keep chickens happy is to build a run or let them out to forage in a safe place. Always check for signs of ill health or external parasites. Covering their run to stop wild birds from entering can prevent some diseases.

Disease Management

If a chicken gets sick, they should be isolated from the flock as soon as possible. New birds should be quarantined before being introduced to the old flock. If you have taken birds to the exhibition areas, you should check them for external parasites and hold them for a few days to ensure they have not picked up any infections. For severe diseases the vet should be called as soon as possible. Some diseases will also require you to slaughter sick birds.

Chicken Manure Disposal Schedules

Chickens are birds and will poop at will anytime. This means that even if they are sleeping they will make a mess. This requires clean up on a daily basis. One of the easiest ways to manage this is to place some shelves below the roosts and put the poop into the compost by simply cleaning the shelves.

Printed in Germany
by Amazon Distribution
GmbH, Leipzig

17902600R00050